The Truth about Ebola: What You Need to Know to Prepare for & Survive a Global Pandemic

Written by Eric Anderson

This book contains material protected under International and Federal Copyright Laws and Treaties. Any unauthorized reprint or use of this material is prohibited. No part of this book may be reproduced or transmitted in any form or by any means, electronic or mechanical, including photocopying, recording, or by any information storage and retrieval system without express written permission from the author.

© 2014 All rights reserved.

Disclaimer:

The information contained in this book is for general information purposes only.

While we endeavor to keep the information up to date and correct, we make no representations or warranties of any kind, express or implied, about the completeness, accuracy, reliability, suitability or availability with respect to the book or the information, products, services, or related graphics contained in the book for any purpose. Any reliance you place on such information is therefore strictly at your own risk.

None of the information in this this book is meant to be construed as medical advice. Always consult with a medical profession prior to making any changes that could impact your health.

Ebola is not something to be taken lightly. If you have reason to believe you have Ebola or someone you know has Ebola, immediate medical attention is required.

Contents

Introduction	6
A Brief History of Ebola	9
Where Is Ebola Now?	11
How Bad Is Ebola?	14
How Does It Spread?	16
Signs and Symptoms of Ebola	19
Diagnosis	21
Stopping Ebola in Its Tracks: Contact Tracing	22
Is There a Cure for Ebola?	24
What Could Ebola Become?	25
Precautions to Take When Infection Is of Concern	27
What to Do If You Suspect You Have Ebola	30
A Brief Note Regarding the Rest of the Book	32
What to Do If There's an Outbreak	34
When Should You Lock Down?	37
Locking Down: No One In or Out	40
Stocking Up: The Supplies You Should Have On Hand	42
Water	44
Food: The Survival Pantry	49
Shelter, Light & Heat	52
Communication	54

Emergency Medical Kit	55
Other Supplies	58
Back-Up Supplies	60
The Sick Room	62
Protection	66
Choosing a Secondary Retreat	69
The Bug Out Bag	73
Body Disposal	75
Addendum I: Another Infection in New York	77

Introduction

The **Ebola virus**, also known as **Ebola hemorrhagic fever**, is a deadly virus that kills the majority of people who contract it. Anyone who has done even a little research into this nefarious disease knows just how scary it is. Death from Ebola is a painful affair as your body hemorrhages uncontrollably both inside and out.

It's caused by one of four viruses in the *Ebolavirus genus*. The viruses known to cause Ebola in in humans are the *Bundibugyo virus* (BDBV), the *Sudan virus* (SUDV), the *Tai Forest virus* (TAFV) and a virus known simply as the *Ebola virus* (EBOV). The latter is the most sinister of the group and is the virus currently tearing through multiple countries in West Africa. There's a fifth virus in the genus known as the *Reston virus* (RESTV), but it's limited to animals and no humans have been documented with this virus, to date.

The host animal of the Ebola virus isn't known for sure, but a number of scientists believe it's the fruit bat. The virus affects both animals and humans and can be passed from infected mammals to humans when they come in contact with contaminated animal corpses, blood or body fluids. Many of the Ebola outbreaks in Africa are believed to be attributed to the butchering and consumption of contaminated bush meat, which comes from animals like bats, cheetahs and other animals native to Africa.

The virus thus far has largely been contained to the African nations where outbreaks have been occurring since its discovery. While most previous outbreaks occurred in remote areas of the jungle and were easy to contain, the most recent outbreak is taking place in a populated urban area of West Africa and is the worst outbreak seen thus far. Overwhelmed medical facilities are hotbeds for the virus as it's passed from person to person in the hospital and by those who come in close contact with sick individuals. Thousands have died and tens of thousands more could end up dying before the disease runs its course.

The fear of Ebola has led many people to turn to the Internet to research the disease, and there are a number of sites disseminating false information that's designed to get headlines and draw attention, but the information being given is questionable at best. While there may be a shred of truth to some of the articles, the reality is often far from what's being portrayed. This book was created to present the known facts on Ebola in a form that's easy to read and has been condensed into one location where much of the information you need to know is available.

It also contains advice on what could be done from a prepper's standpoint to prepare for the coming of the virus should it make the jump across the ocean and not get contained before it starts spreading. There has only been one small outbreak in the United States so far and it appears to have been contained before any additional infections took place, so now is not the time to start panicking. Now, however, is the best time to start preparing in case things do take a turn for the worse and virus makes the jump across the ocean and we start seeing larger outbreaks.

You can never start preparing for a pandemic situation too early and you can never be too prepared.

Chances are you'll never have to use your emergency stockpile or your training, but it's better to have the supplies and not need them than to end up needing them and not have them. One thing's for certain...If you wait until it's obvious you need to start gathering supplies, everyone else will be doing the same. You aren't going to be able to get the gear you need and you'll be left to fight over what little scraps you can find.

A Brief History of Ebola

The Ebola virus was first discovered when dual outbreaks occurred in the Democratic Republic of the Congo and Sudan in 1976. It's named after the Ebola River, which is located near the village in the Congo where the disease was first discovered. 53% of the 284 people infected in the initial outbreak in Sudan died, while 88% of the 318 people infected in the Democratic Republic of the Congo succumbed to the disease. It spread mainly through close personal contact with infected patients and through use of contaminated needles in hospitals. Another outbreak occurred in 1979 in the same area of South Sudan as the first outbreak. Like the first outbreak, the culprit was the Sudan virus and 22 out of 34 people who contracted the virus died.

Fast forward to the 1990's and Ebola begins to appear in other nations due to infected monkeys being transported to facilities in Italy, the Philippines and the United States. 7 total people showed signs of being infected but never contracted the disease.

From 1994 to 1996, there were 6 more outbreaks in Africa. Here they are in chronological order:

- In 1994, 31 of 52 (60%) patients died in an Ebola virus outbreak in Gabon.
- Also in 1994, a single patient along the Ivory Coast contracted the Tai Forest virus and survived. This case was related to contact with a chimpanzee corpse.

- A major outbreak occurred in the Democratic Republic of the Congo in 1995. 250 of 315 (81%) infected patients died as the Ebola virus spread through contact with family members and hospitals.
- Another major outbreak occurred in 1996, with 21 of 37 (57%) of infected patients dying in an Ebola outbreak in Gabon. This outbreak was attributed to contact with and the subsequent butchering of a chimpanzee corpse.
- Another outbreak occurred in Gabon later in the same year, this time killing 45 out of 60 (74%) who contracted the virus.
- One of the medical professionals treating the Gabon outbreak traveled to South Africa and carried the disease into Johannesburg. The scientist and the nurse who cared for him were infected with Ebola. The scientist lived and the nurse died.

Additional outbreaks have occurred in the Congo in 2007 and 2008, Uganda in 2011 and 2012, the Congo again in 2012, and Uganda again near the end of 2012. More than 225 total deaths occurred as a result of these outbreaks.

While some of the aforementioned outbreaks in Africa resulted in a large number of deaths, they were largely contained to small areas in the country where they occurred. It wasn't until the recent outbreak that infections accelerated rapidly and are showing no signs of slowing down.

Where Is Ebola Now?

The current outbreak of the Ebola virus started in March 2014 and widespread transmission of the disease is taking place in Guinea, Liberia and Sierra Leone. It's the worst outbreak seen thus far and is threatening to break out of Africa and makes its way to the rest of the world. To date, nearly 9,000 cases have been reported. Of the reported cases, nearly 4,500 patients have died from the disease. By the time you read this, there will undoubtedly have been more cases and more deaths due to the Ebola virus. This chapter has had to be amended three times while the book was being written to account for new cases.

Cases popped up briefly in Nigeria and Senegal, but the disease has been contained in both of those areas. Spain also had a single case of Ebola make it across their borders, but it was contained quickly.

It's estimated that the infection rate could climb to as many as 10,000 cases per week within a couple months if efforts to stop Ebola aren't stepped up. The current outbreak has already infected and killed more people than all previous outbreaks combined and it's showing no sign of letting up. In fact, by almost all accounts, it appears to be gaining a full head of steam.

As far as the rest of the world goes, there have been 3 recent cases that made headlines in Dallas, Texas. The first case occurred when a man flew from Liberia to Dallas on September 20th, 2014, and went to the hospital 5 days later when he fell ill. It isn't clear whether the man knew he had Ebola when he boarded the plane from Africa. The hospital in Dallas misdiagnosed the case after the first visit, sending the man home with antibiotics. He returned to the hospital on the 28th of September, at which time it was confirmed he had Ebola. The second case came about as a nurse who was treating the first patient was infected, even though precautions were taken and protective gear was worn during treatment. It isn't known exactly how the nurse contracted the disease during the course of treating the first patient, but it's suspected proper safety protocol wasn't followed.

As this book was getting ready to go to press, a third case popped up in the United States. This third case was another of the nurses who treated the infected patient.

The current small outbreak in the U.S. has raised some eyebrows because the United States has been bringing infected U.S. citizens who are infected abroad back to U.S. soil for treatment. The patients are treated in isolation and protective gear is worn, but the fact that these nurses contracted Ebola while supposedly wearing protective gear has to be of utmost concern. It's likely there was some breach of protocol that caused the infections, but that's all speculation at this point. For now, it's sometime to watch closely to make sure it's been contained.

This current small outbreak in the United States isn't much to be worried about (unless you came in contact with one of the infected people), but it is something that needs to be monitored closely. As long as a rash of new cases don't start popping up, no action other than preparing for a local outbreak is required.

At press time, reports were coming in that the United States is beginning to quarantine travelers from stricken nations in an attempt to prevent them from bringing Ebola into the country and infecting others. This is a step in the right direction and may be enough to stop Ebola from entering the U.S. should this policy be enforced across the board.

How Bad Is Ebola?

For many of those unlucky enough to contract it, Ebola is a deadly disease.

Past outbreaks of Ebola have seen anywhere from 25% to 90% fatality rates amongst people who contract the virus and the current outbreak has killed more than half of the people it's infected. By all accounts, Ebola is a dangerous and potentially-deadly disease and it's one for which no cure and no real treatment exists.

To be fair, most experts agree the death rate from Ebola would be drastically lower in an outbreak in a developed nation, as the quality of care afforded each patient would be much better than what's given in Africa. The sooner it's caught and the better care that's received upon contraction, the better the chance of survival becomes. The exact death rate that would be realized isn't known, but it's safe to say Ebola is a still a potentially-deadly disease, no matter where it's contracted.

Once the virus infects the human body, it begins replicating itself and traveling in the blood, damaging and destroying organs it comes in contact with and weakening the immune system along the way. The vast majority of deaths due to ebola come about as the virus lowers the ability of the body to form blood clots, causes organs to fail and reduces the ability of the immune system to respond to infection, which leads to sepsis and, ultimately, death.

By all accounts, death from Ebola is a tortuous and painful ordeal. It can take up to a couple weeks from the time symptoms show up for a patient to either die or recover. Recovery is a relative term because, while the virus may no longer exist in the patient and antibodies will have formed that prevent future infection, the damage incurred during the infection may cause problems that stick with the patient for the rest of their life.

How Does It Spread?

It isn't known exactly which animals are natural hosts for the Ebola virus, but it's thought to have come from fruit bats. The cause of an outbreak isn't always known, but it's suspected that most outbreaks are caused by the first human host(s) coming in contact with an infected animal. Subsequent cases are transmitted by the infected human(s) to others around them.

Once the Ebola virus comes in contact with a mucous membrane or break in the skin, it fuses itself to the exposed cells in that area. The virus then begins replicating itself and releasing more of the virus into the infected person's system. As the virus spreads, symptoms will start to occur, but it can take up to 21 days for the infection to become outwardly apparent.

The virus can be spread in a variety of ways, including the following:

- **Direct contact with broken skin or mucous membranes like the eyes, nose or mouth of an infected patient.**
- **Contact with blood from an infected patient.**
- **Contact with the body fluids of an infected patient, including feces, urine, sweat, saliva and semen.** Ebola can hide in semen for up to 3 months after a patient has recovered.
- **Contact with an infected animal or the body fluids of an infected animal.**
- **Eating an infected animal.**

While Ebola isn't considered an airborne virus, coughing and sneezing can spray particles of Ebola into the air that may settle on items nearby. If an infected patient coughs or sneezes close enough to someone and the virus comes in contact with their mucous membranes, that person could conceivably contract the virus. While most sources state Ebola isn't an *airborne* virus, there are a handful of experts who have stated it may be transmissible through *aerosol* particles. What this means is there is the potential for a cough, vomiting or even the flushing of a toilet to create particles of infected matter that could be inhaled or could land on clean surfaces and contaminate them.

Here's a link to an interesting commentary from the Center for Infectious Disease Research and Policy at the University of Minnesota:

http://www.cidrap.umn.edu/news-perspective/2014/09/commentary-health-workers-need-optimal-respiratory-protection-ebola

Ebola can live for several hours outside the body, so there's no telling whether a surface is contaminated or not. When traveling in an area where an outbreak is underway, it's best to assume everything is contaminated and act accordingly. Don't leave the house without full protective gear, including a face shield, gloves, a body suit and shoe covers. While most sources state an N95 mask is sufficient protection, the article above states "The minimum level of protection in high-risk settings should be a respirator with an assigned protection factor greater than 10."

The vast majority of transmitted cases come when patients get sick and health care practitioners and family members come in close contact with them and their infected body fluids. Failure to wear the proper safety attire could result in the disease rapidly spreading to others. Sometimes, the disease can spread even when precautions are taken, as was the case in Texas. A small slip-up can result in contraction of the disease.

While Ebola is contagious, it isn't thought to be transmissible through food or through water and it isn't believed to be an airborne virus. A small number of cases have reportedly come about as a result of handling contaminated bushmeat, but Ebola is unlikely to be transmitted via the regular food supply in developed countries.

Ebola is highly-contagious if you come in contact with infected body fluids, but that's pretty much the only way it can be spread as it stands now. Hospitals across the Western World are prepared to handle Ebola patients and there are specially-trained teams poised at the ready to strike each and every time a case is announced. It's unlikely Ebola will spread across the United States in its current form.

Signs and Symptoms of Ebola

While it's currently highly unlikely anyone in any nation other than the African nations previously listed will develop Ebola, it's possible an outbreak could occur due to a patient traveling outside of Africa after contracting the disease. We saw this recently with the patient who traveled from Africa to Dallas before he started showing signs of being ill. The outbreak was contained quickly and it appears only two other people were infected before the patient passed away at the hospital.

To date, most cases of Ebola have been confined to Africa, so there isn't much concern of getting infected unless you've traveled to one of the impacted African nations recently and are starting to show signs of infection. Family members of patients and the health care providers tasked with caring for them are at the highest risk because they're the ones most likely to come in contact with infected body fluids.

If an outbreak occurs near you, the following signs may be indicative that you've been infected with the virus:

- **Bad headache.**
- **Diarrhea.**
- **Fever over 101.5° that won't break.**
- **Hemorrhaging from the ears, eyes, nose and mouth.**
- **Impaired liver and kidney function.**
- **Internal hemorrhaging.**
- **Muscle aches and pains.**

- **Muscle weakness and fatigue.**
- **Sore throat.**
- **Stomachache.**
- **Unexplained bruising.**
- **Vomiting.**

The symptoms of Ebola usually occur within 8 to 10 days of infection, but the disease can incubate for up to 21 days before symptoms show up.

Many of the symptoms are nonspecific to Ebola and can come about as a result of colds, flus and other illnesses that are nowhere near as deadly as Ebola. However, early detection of Ebola is absolutely critical, so get yourself checked out immediately if you're showing signs of infection and have reason to believe you've been in close contact with someone who has the virus.

Diagnosis

Ebola symptoms can be similar to the flu, so diagnosis in the early stages can be difficult. In some cases, infected patients have been sent home because the hospital didn't make the diagnosis right away.

If a patient is displaying signs of Ebola and has been in an area where the disease is prevalent or has been in contact with an infected person, the patient should be hospitalized. The patient should be isolated at the hospital and further tests should be performed.

There are a number of laboratory tests that can be given to diagnose Ebola. Diagnosis of patients who have only been infected for a short time and haven't yet started to show signs of infection is difficult. Once symptoms start to show, diagnosis becomes easier and there are a number of blood and lab tests that can be performed to determine whether Ebola is the cause of the symptoms. The most accurate test is the polymerase chain reaction (PCR) test, which checks for the virus' genetic signature. This test can be used to detect Ebola when very little Ebola is present in the body, but may not produce positive results early on in an infection. Other tests look for the antibodies the body produces to battle Ebola, but these tests can take even longer to produce results.

Once a positive diagnosis is made, the authorities in the area need to act fast. The patient should be isolated in the hospital if it hasn't already been done and contact tracing should be performed to identify other potential patients.

Stopping Ebola in Its Tracks: Contact Tracing

Because of its long incubation period and the fact that many patients go undiagnosed while the symptoms are still minor, there's the potential for a number of people to get infected before a patient ever makes his or her way to the hospital.

Every time a new patient is discovered, contact tracing must be performed in order to ensure all infected people are quarantined and hospitalized before they can infect others. Contact tracing means searching out and locating everyone the patient came in direct contact with while he or she was contagious. This is relatively easy when only 1 or 2 patients in an area have contracted the disease. It gets infinitely harder when there are multiple patients who have to be traced.

Here's why…Say you have 1 patient with Ebola who comes in direct contact with 20 people who haven't been infected. Locating those 20 people and monitoring them for signs of Ebola would be fairly easy. Now, say you find 2 more people who have been infected in that group of 20 and each of them came in contact with an average of 20 people. You now have a total of 60 people who have potentially been infected. You've got the 20 from the first group and 40 from the second group, assuming there's no overlap between the groups. Let's now say you find 4 more cases in the current group of people. If those 4 cases each came in contact with an average of 20 people each, there are 80 new people who have to be tracked down and monitored. Add those to the people who are already being monitored and you've got 160 people who have to be monitored. As you can see, the numbers grow exponentially once you've got a few people who are infected and the disease can spiral out of control.

Contact tracing seeks to find and isolate new cases as quickly as possible, before they have the chance to infect anyone else. As soon as signs of infection appear, the patients are isolated and treated, so no new contacts can be infected.

What you need to take from all this is that if officials contact you and start asking you questions about symptoms of Ebola, there's a pretty good chance you've been in contact with a patient who has the disease. Find out who that patient is and assess how closely you were in contact with him or her. Even if the officials that interview you don't quarantine you, it might be a good idea to isolate yourself and avoid close contact with others until you can be sure you don't have the disease.

Is There a Cure for Ebola?

While there are vaccines and experimental drugs in the works, testing takes a long time and there are currently no vaccines that will protect you against the Ebola virus or any drugs that will cure you if you do contract it.

Early detection and hospitalization is critical, as there are a handful of things the hospital can do to help. Most hospitals provide intravenous fluids and balancing salts to ill patients in an attempt to make sure they're getting the nutrients and liquids they need in order to survive. Much of the current treatment for Ebola is really nothing more than watching for new symptoms and treating them as they occur. Maintaining a good oxygen supply and ensuring the patients vital signs are in good shape can help doctors and nurses identify new issues early on.

A patient's chances of survival are largely dependent on the ability of the patient's immune system to fight off the disease before too much damage is dealt to vital organs. Hospitalized patients are monitored for signs of organ failure and are treated for symptoms as they arise. Medical care in the Western world is superior to the care afforded patients in Africa, so the death rate from Ebola should it make the jump to the Western world isn't expected to be as high.

Once a patient has recovered from Ebola, it's unlikely that patient will contract it again. Antibodies are developed that can last 10 years or longer.

What Could Ebola Become?

The World Health Organization (WHO) has estimated the current outbreak can be contained in as little as 6 months, but not all virologists and scientists are on-board with this estimate. Some are going on record as stating Ebola may never be contained. In a recent bbc.com article, a virologist at the University of Nottingham called the situation "desperate" and said the virus now has the opportunity to adapt to thrive in people due to the large number of cases that have occurred this time around.

Here's a link to the article:

http://www.bbc.com/news/health-29060239

If the virus mutates and adapts to its human hosts, it could become even more virulent and start spreading at a faster rate. If that happens, all bets are off. While it's accelerating rapidly in Africa due to lack of good medical care, a mutation could make it more virulent and cause it to spread world-wide.

There's also a chance Ebola could mutate into an airborne virus, which by all accounts would be very, very bad. Here's a link to an article on CNN.com about the possibility of Ebola going airborne:

http://www.cnn.com/2014/09/12/health/ebola-airborne/

Right now, the only way to contract Ebola is to come in direct contact with infected body fluids. If Ebola changes as it replicates, and there's evidence it's a sloppy replicator and is prone to genetic mutation, it could become an airborne virus. If this happens, the virus could spread in a manner similar to the common cold and something as simple as a cough or a sneeze could transmit it to others. While Ebola is unlikely to spread unchecked in the United States in its current form, a mutation could make current efforts to control and contain the disease completely ineffective.

Every time a new person is infected and passes it on to others, there's a chance the disease could mutate. If it mutates into an airborne virus, it could quickly spiral out of control and millions might die instead of the thousands that are currently dying from Ebola. A single person on an airplane could infect the entire plane. The infected people would then head home, infecting everyone they come in contact with as the disease spread unchecked throughout the general population. It would take some time for officials to realize Ebola had gone airborne, and by the time they figured it out, it might have spread so wide it couldn't be stopped.

A disease tearing through the world at this rate would break down all normal forms of commerce and communication. The only way to ensure survival would be to isolate yourself from the rest of the world and ride it out. Even then, that might not be enough.

To be clear, this hasn't happened yet and there's no evidence indicating it's going to happen. It's just a theory being tossed around by infectious disease experts at this point. However, if you hear Ebola has gone airborne, it's time to start paying close attention to all new developments and to consider locking down inside your home.

Precautions to Take When Infection Is of Concern

For those who are traveling to an area where there's risk of contracting Ebola or if you're in an area where an outbreak occurs, there are some precautions you can take to help ensure you don't contract the disease. Following these precautions won't guarantee you won't get infected, but they'll help tilt the odds in your favor.

Here are the precautions you should follow:

- **Wash your hands and arms with soap and water regularly.**
- **If you suspect you've come in contact with something that's infected, wash yourself immediately with soap and water or an alcohol-based hand sanitizer.**
- **Keep any openings or breaks in your skin covered.**
- **Avoid contact with the body fluids of other people.**
- **Avoid personal contact like handshakes, hugs, kisses and sexual contact.**
- **Don't touch clothing or bedding that may have been in contact with an infection person.**
- **Don't touch people who have been infected.** This includes dead bodies that may be infected.
- **Avoid contact with animals that could be infected.**
- **Don't handle or eat bushmeat.**

- **Steer clear of facilities (hospitals, doctor's offices, etc.) where infected people may congregate.**
- **Avoid public transportation in areas where an outbreak has occurred.**
- **Incinerate laundry and clothing that has come in contact with an infected person.**

Health care workers and people who are in close contact with Ebola patients need to take extra care to ensure they aren't infected. This includes wearing protective gear and avoiding direct contact with infected people, body fluids from infected people and the bodies of people who have died from Ebola.

The following gear is commonly worn by those on the front lines fighting this deadly disease:

- Medical mask.
- Surgical cap.
- Respirator.
- Goggles.
- Overalls.
- Scrubs.
- Apron.
- Double gloves.
- Boots.

It's important that all areas of the skin are covered and there is no exposed skin that could come in contact with the virus. Precautions should be taken when taking gear off to make sure the exposed areas of the gear don't come in contact with the skin.

Patients who are displaying signs of Ebola should be immediately isolated from other patients. If you suspect you or someone you know has been infected, the only place you should travel is to your local hospital. Call ahead and explain the situation, so you can ensure proper protocol is followed. If you're in a foreign country, contact your country's embassy or consulate for instructions on where you should go and how you should get there.

What to Do If You Suspect You Have Ebola

Let me begin this chapter by stating the chances of you contracting Ebola outside of the areas of West Africa where the current outbreak is taking place are slim to none. In recent years, only a couple people have contracted the disease in the United States and both were nurses who were in close contact with a patient who caught the disease while in Africa. That could change in the future, but for now, the chances of you having Ebola are extremely slim.

If you've been watching news reports and researching Ebola online and are convinced you might have Ebola, you aren't alone. The CDC is getting hundreds of calls per day from people just like you who are afraid they've been infected. The vast majority of these calls are false alarms.

If you or a loved one has recently traveled to an affected area of Africa or have reason to believe you've come in contact with someone who is infected, it's important you contact your doctor right away. If you're in the United States, it's a good idea to also contact the Center for Disease control and explain your concerns to them. They'll tell you the best course of action to take, but you're going to have to be patient. They field a lot of calls and may not seem as concerned that you have Ebola as you are.

Once you've contacted your physician and the CDC, they should give you instructions you need to follow. If they're concerned you're infected, they'll tell you where to go and how you should get there. It's important you seek medical care. Ebola isn't something you can ride out at home. You have a much better chance of survival when you're being provided medical care than you do if you were to stay home and try to tough it out. Don't show up at your doctor's office or the local ER unannounced. If you do have Ebola, they're going to need time to prepare to take you in and if you walk in on your own, the chances of you infecting others increases tenfold.

If you get checked out by a doctor and are given a clean bill of health and you're still concerned, keep a close watch for signs and symptoms the virus is spreading through your body. A temperature over 100° F, severe headaches, muscle and joint pain, gastrointestinal distress and vomiting are all symptoms of Ebola. Unexplained bruising and bleeding that won't stop are signs of the more advanced stages of Ebola.

A Brief Note Regarding the Rest of the Book

Much of what you're going to read in the rest of the book assumes a worst-case scenario regarding the Ebola virus. It contains information that could potentially be used to survive a large local outbreak of Ebola and is good information to have on hand. At this point in time, there is no need to panic and lock yourself in your home unless you're currently residing in West Africa near an area where an outbreak is occurring.

Now is the time to prepare for a local Ebola outbreak. The chances of an outbreak actually happening near you are very, very slim, but it's best to be prepared to take immediate action should one occur. The situation could progress from bad to worse very, very quickly in certain worst-case scenarios and you don't want to be caught completely unprepared. By the time you realize you need survival supplies and food, everyone else will have realized the same thing. Gather your supplies and food now and you'll be able to stay two steps ahead of the rest of the pack in the unlikely event the disease makes the jump to Western world and starts to spread.

Whatever you do, don't get yourself worked into a panic over Ebola.

Yes, a couple people in the United States have been infected by a patient who contracted the disease in Africa and flew to Dallas. The two people (to date) who were infected were nurses who were in daily contact with the sick person and were exposed to all sorts of body fluids.

Vomit, blood, urine and feces from the infected person were all part of their daily routine. They were wearing protective gear, but there are reports coming from the hospital that indicate proper protocol may not have been followed. It helps to remember that the infected nurses and the sick man came in contact with hundreds, if not thousands, of other people in the Dallas area and nobody else has shown signs of infection.

Is the Ebola virus scary? Absolutely. The best-case scenario for those contracting it is a slow and painful recovery from a disease that can do lasting damage. Is it time to panic and lock yourself in your house? No, but by all means watch what's going on both at home and in the rest of the world.

You can never be too prepared and you can never be too informed.

What to Do If There's an Outbreak

While there haven't been any major flare-ups yet outside of Africa, it's feared an outbreak could be caused by a sick person traveling from Africa to another country, infecting people on the plane and others they come in contact with once they arrive at their destination. Anyone who comes in close contact with a sick person once symptoms appear is at risk and may be infected. The problems lies in the fact that Ebola doesn't always present itself in the same manner and you can't tell someone has Ebola just by looking at them.

When an outbreak is underway, your best bet is to avoid human contact as much as possible. Steer clear of places where large numbers of people gather like sporting events, schools, shopping centers and restaurants. The problem doesn't lie so much in the people around you since you're unlikely to catch Ebola from someone you aren't within a few feet of. The bigger issue is the many surfaces that might be harboring the disease. All it takes is for an infected person to cough or sneeze and spray spittle on a surface and anyone who comes in contact with it is at risk of contracting Ebola.

Here's a list of just some of the places you should avoid:

- **Airplanes.**
- **Concerts.**
- **Libraries.**
- **Malls.**
- **Nightclubs and bars.**
- **Parties.**

- **Public buildings.**
- **Public transportation.**
- **Public transportation.**
- **Restaurants.**
- **Schools.**
- **Sporting events.**
- **Stores.**

Basically, if people gather there, you don't want to be there. You're going to want to isolate yourself and have as little contact with the outside world as possible. If an outbreak gets bad enough, you may find the area you're living in is placed under forced quarantine or curfew. The authorities will restrict when and where people are allowed to move about in order to avoid further contact with others. If a forced curfew is announced, that means things are spiraling out of control and it's time to either lock down or get out of town.

The length of time you're going to need to isolate yourself from outside contact varies depending on a number of factors, first and foremost being how bad the infection is and how widespread it's become. It's going to be worse in a big city where there are more people to spread the disease around to than in a small town. It's also going to depend on how many people the patient came in close contact with and how many others were infected.

If it's an isolated case or two in your area, as was the case in Dallas, you probably don't need to isolate yourself. Life will continue on without you and you'll end up losing your job and alienating yourself and your children for no good reason. On the other hand, if you're hearing reports the disease is spreading quickly, it's time to consider hunkering down and riding out the storm. If nobody in your house is infected when you lock down, the chances of you contracting the disease without coming in contact with an infected person are slim to none.

Use this knowledge to your advantage to minimize risk.

When Should You Lock Down?

The decision to lock down is something that can't be taken lightly.

You're going to have to stop going to work and cut off face-to-face contact with the outside world. Start saving up sick time and money now, so you're prepared if you have to take an extended leave of absence. If you have children, you're going to have to pull them out of school and you may be forced to explain to local authorities why you're making the decisions you're making. It helps to remember that, in the end, it's up to you when you go into lockdown and nobody else should be allowed to make that decision for you.

You don't want to go into lockdown unnecessarily, but you also don't want to wait until it's too late. I've set the rule that if there's an outbreak within 50 miles of my home or place of work, I'm going to lock down until the virus has been contained. For smaller outbreaks like the one that occurred recently in Dallas, that could be a couple days. If the virus becomes more virulent or it appears to have gone airborne, I'm going to lockdown if it's within 250 miles. I'll remain in lockdown until I'm positive it's been contained.

Is this overkill? Maybe, but I'm of the opinion it's best to err on the side of caution. Here are some of the warning signs to look for that may indicate an Ebola outbreak is imminent in your area:

- **You start seeing more frequent reports about Ebola outbreaks in your country of residence**

and it looks like the authorities are having trouble containing the outbreaks.
- **Larger numbers of infections per outbreak is also a sign things are starting to get worse.**
- **Officials are hitting the news circuits telling everyone to remain calm even though the facts don't seem to support what they're saying.**
- **If a state of emergency is declared, it's time to lockdown until it's lifted.** You may be forced to lock down regardless, but at least you'll be able to shelter in place with the supplies you've gathered.
- **Cases are popping up in your state or in nearby cities and they appear to be getting closer.**
- **Stores are beginning to run out of food and emergency supplies.** If you wait until this happens, it may be too late to gather the supplies you need.
- **Panicked people are showing up in your area asking for help and shelter.**

If the rule of law breaks down in your area and you live in a populated city or even a town with a decent amount of people, you may want to consider getting out of town and heading to a secondary location that's less-populated. It's best to get out of town sooner rather than later because in a truly lawless situation roadblocks may be set up and you'll have a target painted on your back as you're trying to get out of town.

Invest in a police scanner and familiarize yourself with how to use it, so you can monitor how bad the situation is getting outside. If there are signs the police force is on the verge of being overwhelmed or, even worse, if the police scanner goes completely silent, it's time to start considering your options.

Locking Down: No One In or Out

If an Ebola outbreak occurs locally and it reaches the point where you have to go into lockdown, it's best to do so sooner rather than later. The more time family members spend out and about, the more likely it becomes they'll be exposed to an infected person.

Once you make the decision to lock down, nobody leaves or enters until the all-clear has been given. Every time someone who hasn't been infected with the virus leaves the house, there's the potential that person could return with the virus and infect the rest of the people in the house. While the chances of someone leaving and coming back with the virus are relatively slim, locking down ensures nobody brings Ebola into the home, so it's a must that nobody leaves. It's also a must that you don't let anyone new in once you make the decision to lock down.

If someone does leave and you want to let them back in or you want to let someone else in who has had contact with the outside world, they're going to need to be isolated and watched for at least 21 days. If they don't display signs of being sick within 21 days, they aren't likely to be infected and can be allowed to rejoin the rest of the people in the house.

It's important that no one enters or leaves the room they're contained in and no contact is made with the person or any fluids from their body. What this means is all bathing, eating, using the bathroom and anything else that's done by that person needs to be done in the confines of the quarantine room until the quarantine is over. For obvious reasons, it's preferable that the person is quarantined in a room with a bathroom. If you're forced to isolate patients in a room that doesn't have a bathroom, all garbage and waste materials should be disposed of in heavy plastic bags that are wrapped and taped shut before they leave the room. Any contact with vomit, feces or other body materials could result in infection. Bring the trash and waste materials outdoors and incinerate them.

The toughest part of locking down is going to be turning away sick people who show up asking for help. It wouldn't be hard for most of us to turn away a complete stranger, but what if the person on the other side of the door is a close family friend or a relative? Then it becomes much more difficult to turn them away, but you're going to have to be able to do it if you want to maintain a disease-free lockdown.

Stocking Up: The Supplies You Should Have On Hand

While it isn't time to panic or go into hiding, there's no better time than right now to gather the supplies you're going to need to ride out an Ebola outbreak. Even if there is never an Ebola outbreak close enough to your home to warrant locking down, the supplies you're going to gather can be used in the event there's any sort of emergency that cuts you off from the food supply and the rest of the world. While unprepared people will be forced to forage for food and supplies when food and supplies are going to be at their scarcest, you'll be able to stay home and avoid contact with potentially-infected people.

Whatever you do, don't procrastinate until an outbreak occurs. If things go bad in a hurry, there will be a mad rush for supplies and survival gear and stores will be picked clean. Food, water and the basic necessities will be the first to go, followed by guns, ammo and anything else people think they're going to need to ride out the outbreak. Unless you feel like rushing from store to store hoping to pick up a few scraps left behind by others while possibly getting infected by everyone you come in contact with, now's the time to stock up.

People often ask how much supplies they should stock up on. The answer to this question is as much as you can afford. A week's worth of supplies is good. There's a pretty good chance most outbreaks will be contained within a week and you'll be able to return to normal life. A month's worth of supplies will give you some breathing room should an infection take off like it has in Africa. A 3-month supply is even better because it gives you an extra 2 months' worth of food and supplies should the outbreak get worse and start to spiral out of control. If you can afford a 6-month to 1-year supply then by all means, that's the route you should go. Should the Ebola virus go airborne, it could take that long or longer to get it under control, if we're ever able to rein it in.

When stocking up, assume that you're going to have to rely on your survival stockpile for everything. In a bad enough emergency, you could be left without power, water and outside assistance for an extended period of time. While there's a pretty good chance your utilities will continue running unchecked even in the event of an Ebola outbreak, it's best to prepare for a situation in which you don't have access to the basic necessities you're used to having. If electricity, water and garbage services continue, consider that a bonus. You'll be able to live even more comfortably and your emergency supplies will last longer.

In this day and age of instant electricity and water anytime we want it, it's going to take some getting used to it if your utilities suddenly stop working, but it isn't going to be a matter of life and death if you're properly prepped. The basic necessities you need to survive aren't going to change if the infrastructure breaks down.

Water

To put it simply, you aren't going to survive without water. If you fail to put away enough water and you run out, you're going to have to leave your home to find it. This opens you up to exposure to Ebola, robbery and any of a number of other occurrences that probably wouldn't happen if you're able to stay locked up tight in your home and ride out the infection.

You're going to need at least a couple quarts of water per person per day for drinking. If it's hot and the power is out, you're going to need even more water to account for the water lost to sweating. You're going to need roughly double the amount you need for drinking when sanitation and water for cooking are taken into account. This equates to approximately a gallon of water per person per day for each adult member of your household. Young children will need less, but it's important you put enough away for them as well. Don't forget your pets. They're going to need water, too.

The problem with storing enough water to last through an extended emergency is that storing takes up a lot of space. Think of a gallon carton of milk. A family of four is going to need four of those per day. A one week supply for a family of four would require finding room to store the equivalent of 28 milk jugs full of water. A month-long supply of water would take 120 gallon milk jugs. Thinking of saving a 6-month supply of water? Better have space for 720 milk jugs. It's tough to even fathom finding space to store enough water to last through an extended emergency. Of course you can save some space by saving the water in larger containers or drums, but you're still going to need more room than most people have.

The water you do store should be stored in clean, non-corrosive containers that are kept in a cool, dark place. If you're storing the water in milk jugs or water bottles, be aware the plastic is permeable and storing them in the garage near gasoline or other chemicals may result in the water taking up some of the vapors from these chemicals. It's best to store your water in food grade containers, but the cost could be prohibitive. Large water storage drums are available, but they're expensive and difficult to take with you if you have to leave your location in a hurry. If you decide to go this route, it's a good idea to have a supply of water in smaller containers available in addition to the larger drums. High Density Polyethylene containers are the only plastic containers you should use because other types of plastic could leach chemicals into the water.

Make sure you sanitize your storage containers before keeping water in them. Wash them with dishwashing soap and then sanitize them using a solution made by combining a teaspoon of bleach with a couple quarts of water. Rinse the container thoroughly before storing water in it.

Rotate your water supply every 4 to 6 months to ensure it stays fresh.

There may come a time when you run out of stored water and your access to water from your local utility company is either cut off or the water that's being provided is contaminated. Make sure you know where your water intake valve is and shut the water off using the valve as soon as you hear of contamination. Use the remaining uncontaminated water that's in your pipes to fill the bathtubs and sinks in your house. There are inexpensive water storage systems available that will allow you to fill a tub with up to 100 gallons of fresh water.

As long as you got to the shut-off valve in time, your hot water heater will also be full of clean water that can be drained out and used. In order to drain your hot water heater, open the drain plug at the bottom and have someone turn on one of the hot water spigots in the house. Turn off the electricity or gas (whichever your heater runs on) before draining the tank. Toilets are another source of water. The water in the tank should be somewhat clean and even the water in the bowl can be sanitized and used.

If you want to collect as much water as possible and you live in a 2-story home, find the lowest water line in your home and place a bucket beneath the spigot. Turn a faucet on that's at a higher location in the house to get the water flowing. Be prepared to collect all the water that drains out. A significant amount of water will be contained within the pipes and you don't want to lose a bunch of it because you didn't have a large enough storage container.

If you live in a house that has a well, make sure you invest in a manual pump that can be used to draw water from the well if the power grid shuts down. This alone could give you enough water to last through an emergency as long as the groundwater isn't contaminated.

If you have a swimming pool, that's another source of water. There's conflicting information out there on whether saltwater pools have too much salt in them to be considered a safe source of drinking water. I'd say it's best to assume they aren't unless you plan on desalinating the water.

You can also collect rainwater in pots, pans and any other containers you may have on hand. If you want to go bigger, rainwater collection systems are available that can be used to collect rainwater and store it in large drums. Make sure you're up to speed on your local laws because collecting rainwater has been outlawed in some areas.

At some point, you might need to start collecting water from sources that may not be safe for consumption. If there's any question as to the safety of the water, it's best to treat it. Water collected from toilets, swimming pools, rain gutters, ponds, lakes and rivers are all of questionable quality and will need to be treated before you use it. Remember that just because it looks clean doesn't mean it's free of harmful microorganisms. You can treat water by using the methods below to kill off harmful microorganisms and pathogens, but any heavy metals or chemicals in the water will still be there after the water has been treated.

The following methods can all be used to treat water:

- **Filter cloudy water through a coffee filter or a clean towel.** You may have to filter it a few times before it's clear. This will remove larger particles from the water, but won't make it safe to drink.
- **Boil the water.** Bring the water to a rolling boil for 5 minutes.
- **Bleach.** Add 2 drops of unscented liquid bleach (5% to 6 %) to a quart of water and let it sit for at least 30 minutes.

- **Chlorine tablets.** Follow the manufacturer's instructions for sanitizing water.
- **Filters.** Portable water filters can be used to remove contaminants from water. The type of contaminants you can remove and the amount of water that can be filtered before the filter loses effectiveness varies from filter to filter. Only certain types of filters will work to clean water that's been contaminated.
- **Distillation.** This method involves heating the water up until it becomes steam and collecting the vapor as it condenses back into water. This will eliminate many of the impurities from the water.

There's another option for those who are looking to really make sure they're prepared, but it's an expensive one. Atmospheric water generators are now available that will pull water out of the atmosphere and can generate several gallons of water daily. While these water generators are nice to have, they shouldn't be relied upon as your only source of water. They require electricity to run, which is fine as long as the utilities in your area are up and running. If not, you're going to need a lot of gas to keep a generator running in order to provide power to your water generator.

Food: The Survival Pantry

Next to water, food is the second most important item you're going to need on-hand to ensure survival in the event there's an Ebola outbreak near you. You're going to need a steady supply of food and it should be made up of food your family will want to eat every day. This is where a well-stocked survival pantry comes into play. You should have enough food for at least 6 months and preferably a year.

I see a lot of people buying freeze-dried foods or military rations as their emergency food supply. It's fine to have some of these on-hand in case you have to get out of town in a hurry and need something lightweight and easy to carry, but trust me when I say you aren't going to want to eat this type of food day-in and day-out for months on end if there's an extended emergency. If you think your kids complain about leftovers now, think about how much they're going to complain when you only have two choices and both of them are freeze dried. There are other items you can stockpile to ensure you have a ready supply of healthy food on hand.

You can save money on the exorbitant cost of MREs and freeze dried foods and you'll end up healthier and happier with your meal options if you stock your survival pantry with the following foods:

- **Canned foods like vegetables, fruits, meats, soups and beans.** Canned foods taste better than MREs, they're dense in nutrients and they last a long time. The downside is they're heavy and you probably aren't going to have time to load

your vehicle with canned foods if you have to leave home in a hurry.
- **Dried beans and peas.**
- **Crackers and chips.**
- **Nuts and seeds.**
- **Dry pasta.**
- **Peanut butter.**
- **Whole wheat flour.** White flour is devoid of nutrients. Whole wheat flour is a better option for your survival pantry because it contains more nutrients and is better for you.
- **Seasonings.** While seasonings like salt, pepper and herbs and spices aren't a necessity, you'll be glad you have them.
- **Sugar.**
- **Powdered eggs.**
- **Baking soda and baking powder.** If you plan on having baked goods, these are a necessity.
- **Honey.** It's healthy and can be consumed to provide a quick energy boost.
- **Whole grains like wheat, brown rice and barley.**
- **Dried milk.**
- **Cooking oil.** Unrefined vegetable oils like olive oil and coconut oil are a good choice.
- **Instant potatoes.**
- **Ramen noodles.**
- **Coffee and tea.** You don't have to have this in our survival pantry, but the thought of months without a cup of coffee scares me half to death.

When selecting items to put in your survival pantry, choose items you know your family will eat. There's no use putting away 100 cans of canned pineapple you found on clearance if you know your family hates canned pineapple. Instead, try to select comfort foods you know will get eaten. Start with the list above and add to it as you see fit.

Purchasing a 6-month emergency supply of food all at once will break all but the most robust of grocery budgets. Instead, what you can do is buy a couple extra items each time you go grocery shopping. It doesn't look like much, but if you do this every time you head to the store, you'll have a good supply of food built up in no time at all with a negligible impact to your budget.

In addition to storing food, it's a good idea to have a supply of vegetable seeds on hand in case the situation goes from bad to worse and you have to figure out a long-term survival plan. Visit your local nursery or garden center and talk to an expert in order to determine the vegetable seeds that grow best in your area. If you have a large enough lot, I recommend planting several fruit trees now since they can take 5 years or longer to start producing fruit. A couple trees can provide you with hundreds of pounds of healthy fruit annually once they mature. This fruit, along with any extra vegetables you grow in your garden can be canned or dried and saved for the winter months during which you might not be able to grow crops depending on where you live.

Don't forget your pets. They're also going to need a stockpile of food. You don't want to have to start feeding them out of your stockpile.

Shelter, Light & Heat

Most people don't pay close attention to shelter, light and heat when it comes to building up a survival cache. Many of the items you need aren't items you're likely to have on hand unless you're a camping enthusiast and have a well-stocked supply of camping goods. The items discussed in this chapter are great to have on hand in case a situation arises in which you have to leave your home and head out to a less-populated area for a while.

When considering shelter, light and heat, it's best to prepare for the worst-case scenario of having to head off into the wilderness in the middle of winter. What this means is a person living in the Central Valley of California will have a much different list of supplies than a person living in Wisconsin or Northern Maine. While the person living in California can probably get away with packing light, the person in Wisconsin or Maine is going to need cold-weather gear that'll keep them alive under harsh conditions and even then there are no guarantees.

Even if you're able to stay in your home, it's best to assume you're going to have to survive without power at some point and plan accordingly. While most homes are equipped with electric or gas heating units, what are you going to do if you lose power?

A secondary form of heat that doesn't require being on the grid will be required, especially if you want to stay comfortable under harsh winter conditions. Here's a tip that could keep those of you who don't have a wood-burning fireplace alive in the event of an extended emergency during the winter.

Set up a large outdoor fire pit surrounded by smooth river rocks that aren't too heavy to pick up. Build a fire in the pit and bring the warm rocks indoors to provide some much-needed warmth during the winter.

The following items are all good items to stock up on:

- **An oil heater and the right type of oil to run in it.**
- **Candles.**
- **Flashlights and batteries.**
- **Lanterns and wicks.**
- **Oil lights.**
- **Sleeping bags and tents that are appropriately rated for the cold weather you might experience.**
- **Space blankets.**
- **Thermal underwear.**
- **Warm clothes that will keep you warm under harsh winter conditions.**

Start off with a 3- to 5-day supply and add onto your stockpile from there as you can afford it. Ideally, you're going to want to build up to at least a 6-month supply of the consumable items on the list.

Communication

Cell phones may stop working if the normal communications grid goes down. If this happens, you're going to want to have alternate forms of communication.

Wind-up radios, HAM radios and CB radios may be the only connection you have to the outside world. It's a good idea to keep a couple sets of walkie talkies and batteries to power them with your supplies. If anyone has to leave, they'll be able to maintain contact with the rest of the group. And remember, if a person leaves and returns, they need to go into the sick room and be quarantined for at least 21 days before they rejoin the rest of the group.

Flares and flashing emergency lights are also good items to have on hand because they can be used to signal for help if a rescue crew is nearby and you're in trouble.

Emergency Medical Kit

You're going to need a large first aid kit because you aren't going to want to leave the house when basic first aid is needed. It's up to you whether you buy a large kit or assemble one yourself that's tailored to your family's individual needs.

Here are some of the items you're going to want to include in your first aid kit:

- **A thermometer.**
- **A wound stapler and a staple removal kit.**
- **Activated charcoal.**
- **Adhesive bandages.**
- **Airway rebreather tube kit.**
- **Allergy medications.**
- **Aloe vera.**
- **Antibiotic creams.**
- **Anti-diarrheal medication.**
- **Antiseptic.**
- **Artery forceps.**
- **Burn cream.**
- **Butterfly sutures.**
- **Cotton balls.**
- **Cough medicine.**
- **Decongestants.**
- **Emergency dental kit.**
- **Epipens.**
- **Eyedropper.**
- **Eyewash and eye dressings.**
- **Gauze.**

- Heartburn medication.
- Hydrogen peroxide.
- Ice bags.
- Insect repellent.
- Iodine.
- Ipecac syrup.
- Lidocaine.
- Moleskin.
- Nail clippers.
- Needles and thread.
- Neosporin.
- Non-prescription medications and painkillers.
- Oral antibiotics.
- Prescription medications.
- Q-tips.
- Quick clot gauze.
- Scissors.
- Splints.
- Stethoscope.
- Sunblock.
- **Superglue.** Use superglue to glue wounds and cuts shut.
- Tape.
- Tissues.
- Tweezers.
- Vaseline.
- Vitamins.
- Wooden tongue depressors.

If you wear contacts, you're going to need extra contact lenses, extra cases and a stockpile of solution. Buy an extra pair of glasses and keep them in your emergency stockpile. Don't forget to swap them out with a new pair when you update your prescription. Old glasses from a couple prescriptions ago aren't going to do you much good.

All this medical gear is great to have on hand, but it isn't going to do you a bit of good if you don't know what to do with it when you need it. Invest in a comprehensive field first aid manual and store it with your medical kit, so you'll be able to look up how to take care of a number of ailments and illnesses when outside help isn't an option.

It's also a good idea to take CPR classes and first aid classes, if they're available in your area. You can never be too prepared.

Other Supplies

There are a number of other items you're going to want to have on hand. Here are some of the other supplies you're going to want to have in your survival cache:

- A lighter and fuel.
- A portable toilet.
- A shovel.
- Alcohol.
- Antibacterial hand sanitizer.
- Bleach.
- Books and games for the kids.
- Disposable wipes.
- Duct tape.
- Feminine hygiene supplies (tampons, maxi pads, etc.).
- Fire wood.
- Firestarter.
- Heavy garbage bags.
- Large sealable freezer bags.
- Matches.
- Multi-tool.
- N95 masks.
- Napkins.
- Nitrile gloves.
- Paper towels.
- Plastic sheeting.
- Protective clothing.
- Rope and twine.
- Safety goggles.

- **Safety pins.**
- **Soap.**
- **Toilet paper.**
- **Zip ties.**

If you run out of toilet paper, there are other items that can be used. Leaves from non-irritating plants, coffee filters and strips of cloth can all be used. In a pinch, pages out of your local phone book or sheets of newspaper can also be used.

Those of you with infant children are going to need even more supplies. Formula, diapers, powder, diaper rash cream and wipes should all be stockpiled. It's also a good idea to have cloth diapers on hand and to make sure you know how to use them in case you run out of disposable diapers.

Back-Up Supplies

So, you've spend hundreds, if not thousands or even tens of thousands, of dollars building up an impressive survival cache. You've got all your bases covered and feel like you're ready for anything the world can throw at you. Well, I've got news for you. If all of your gear, food and water are stored in one location, you're woefully unprepared. What are you going to do if something happens and you're cut off from that location? What are you going to do if a forced evacuation is announced and you go to return home and all of the roads into your neighborhood are blocked?

While the chances of you being forcefully removed from your home are slim, there are some pretty good reasons to keep a back-up cache or two of supplies hidden far from your home. For one, what if you're out of town and find out Ebola has hit your city hard? Are you going to want to return to town and risk infection to gather supplies? Probably not, and if you've got a back-up cache, you won't have to. Another good reason is you never know when you'll lose access to your main cache and a back-up cache of supplies could mean the difference between survival and slow death.

While the best place to keep a back-up cache would be in or near a remote cabin or home that you own, there are other options if you don't have the money to buy a "vacation" cabin. You can fill waterproof ammunition containers or even 50-gallon drums with supplies and bury them in a remote location only you know about. I've heard of people burying drums all along their bug-out route in case they have to strike off on foot. This allows them to pack light when they head out because they'll be able to replenish their supplies at each of the back-up caches.

You're going to want your back-up cache to be well-hidden, but not so hidden that you aren't able to find it again. Visit your cache location from time-to-time to check on it and make sure you'll be able to find it in an emergency.

The Sick Room

While you would ideally be able to get sick individuals to the hospital for treatment, the health care system could become so overwhelmed they aren't taking on new patients. If this happens, you're going to want to have a sick room set up. A *sick room*, also known as an *isolation room*, is a room to which people who are showing signs of infection can be quarantined so they don't infect the rest of the group. To be completely honest with you, the best course of action would be to kick sick people out of the house before they infect anyone else, but most people aren't going to be willing to send a close friend or family member off to die, myself included.

The sick room needs to be a separate room in the house. If you have a bedroom that's on the opposite end of the house from the rest of the rooms, choose that room.

Do your best to seal the sick room off from the rest of the house. Tape plastic to the walls outside the room to create an area where people who enter the room wearing protective gear can take the gear off. Be aware that removing protective gear is the time when you're most likely to get infected and take all precautions to ensure you don't come in contact with the outside of the gear while removing it. In a pinch, tarps or heavy sheets of plastic hung on both sides of the door should be sufficient as long as the virus hasn't gone airborne. As soon as someone starts showing signs of infection, they should be quarantined to the sick room. Once the sick person enters the sick room, they shouldn't be allowed to leave until they either recover from the virus or they die.

If it turns out the person is infected with Ebola, at some point the sick person will likely need a caretaker. If you have someone willing to enter the room and act as a caretaker, that person should be covered from head-to-toe in protective gear. Disposable gloves, protective clothing, an N95 mask and shoe and head protection should be worn at all times while in the room. They'll need to be removed immediately once the caretaker leaves the room. Be careful not to touch the exposed surfaces of the clothes that could be contaminated with Ebola. Protective gear should be taken outside and burnt once you're done with it.

The following preventative measures should be put in place to lessen the risk of contamination:

- **Avoid touching your eyes, nose, mouth and genitals when you've recently been in the sick room.**
- **Line the mattress in the sick room with plastic to prevent infected body fluids from soaking into the mattress.**
- **Assume that everything in the room is contaminated.** Items that have to be reused should be sanitized with hot, soapy water or a solution of bleach and water. Disposable items should be removed from the house and incinerated.
- **Use paper plates, plastic cups and disposable silverware that can be thrown away after one use.**

- **Wear protective gear every time you enter the sick room.** Remove it before you trek through the rest of the house.
- **Keep the door closed.**
- **Limit the people who are allowed in the sick room.**

The following items should be stocked in a sick room:

- **A bed. If you have room, more than one bed should be placed in the sick room.**
- **A clothes hamper that's lined with a plastic bag.**
- **A garbage pail.**
- **A portable toilet.**
- **A radio.**
- **A two-way handset.**
- **Bleach.**
- **Cotton balls and Q-tips.**
- **Disposable apron.**
- **Face shield.**
- **Flashlight and lantern.**
- **Garbage bags.**
- **Large resealable plastic bags.**
- **Latex gloves.**
- **Leakproof body bags.**
- **M95 masks.**
- **Medications.**
- **Plastic mattress cover.**
- **Plastic sheets.**

- **Rubbing alcohol.**
- **Shoe covers.**
- **Thermometer.**
- **Toilet paper.**
- **Tyvek suit.**
- **Wipes.**

In the event that someone gets sick and is quarantined in the sick room, that person is not to leave the room until you're sure they're better. Anyone entering the room needs to be wearing full protective gear and the gear should be removed as soon as they leave the room. Everything that leaves the room should either be washed immediately or taken outside and incinerated.

To be clear, as long as medical help is available, a sick room should not be an option for quarantining people showing symptoms of Ebola. Medical care from a medical professional is always the best choice and the sooner you get help, the better off you'll be. Caring for the sick isn't something that should be taken lightly and it should only be attempted as a last resort if outside medical care isn't available.

Protection

If things devolve to the point where you have to lockdown in your home or head to a secondary location, you're going to need protection.

When the necessities of life become scarce, the rule of law could break down. If this happens, all bets are off and you're going to need a way to protect yourself from desperate people looking for the supplies they need to survive. The bigger the city you live in, the more at-risk you are of attack. Normally law-abiding citizens may resort to robbery (or worse) when staring starvation in the face. Since you prepped ahead of time, you'll have a huge bull's eye on your back. The more people there are who know about your survival cache, the bigger the bull's eye is going to be.

As a rule of thumb, don't tell anyone you don't want locking down with you about your survival cache. When supplies run out, everyone who didn't prepare for themselves will come calling, asking for help. You'll either have to let them in or turn them away…and the people you turn away could become desperate and launch an attack. The fewer people there are who know about your survival preparation, the better off you'll be in the long run. That is, unless you want a house full of uninvited guests eating your food and using up your supplies.

All your preparation will be for naught if you don't have the means to ensure your gear, food and water don't fall into the hands of the unprepared. The best form of protection available to the average citizen (at least in America) is firearms. When packs of armed bandits are roaming the city looking for easy victims, the best way to ensure you don't become a victim is being prepared to defend yourself.

There are three types of firearms you're going to want to have on hand:

- **A handgun for mid- to short range protection.** Popular calibers include 9mm, .40 or .45.
- **A shotgun for close range protection.** A 12-gauge shotgun is the best for close range protection.
- **A rifle with a scope for mid- to long-range protection.** Popular calibers include .223 and 30-06. Ammunition for .22 rifles is currently very hard to find, but this is a great caliber to have on hand for hunting small game.

If you can afford it, buy a gun for each able-bodied member of your house, along with several extras in the various popular calibers. Stock up on as much ammunition as you can afford, along with extra magazines that can be filled with ammo and quickly swapped out in the event there's a firefight. I'm of the opinion you can never have too many guns or too much ammo. Even if you end up not needing it for defense, the ammo you've stockpiled will be as good as gold if you need to barter for other goods.

In addition to protecting yourself with firearms, there are a number of steps you can take now to ensure your home is protected if there's an emergency. Automatic flood lights, cameras and motion detectors are all nice, but they'll all be useless if the power grid goes down unless you're able to run a generator or power them with solar power.

Take a quick walk around your home and take note of all the potential paths of entry onto your property and into your home. Fences and thorned bushes can make access to your property difficult. Barred windows or thorned bushes in front of windows will help secure your home from invaders looking to get in and out silently. The biggest threat to your safety occurs once an intruder breaches the perimeter. Each capable person in your house should be properly-trained as to how to handle themselves if there's a home invasion and they should be well-versed in the use of firearms for protection.

Choosing a Secondary Retreat

If things start to go bad in the area you're locked down in, it may become necessary to retreat to a more secluded area. Having a secondary location you can head out to is always a good idea, but it's more important for those living in populated areas. If you live in the epicenter of an outbreak and things go downhill fast, you may have to leave the city and should have a backup plan in place.

The best secondary retreats are in isolated areas that are within an hour or two travel time of the area you're located at. While a few hours may not seem like it's far enough away, you have to balance this with the reality that you're probably going to have to fight your way through gridlocked traffic with everyone else who's trying to flee the disease. Choose a remote location where you're unlikely to come in contact with anyone else and it won't matter that you're still too close for comfort to the outbreak area.

It's entirely possible you could end up spending a significant amount of time living at your secondary retreat, so take extra care to examine both the dwelling and the area around the dwelling closely. Here are some questions to ask while walking the property:

- Is there room to plant seeds and grow crops?
- What is winter going to be like in this area? Will the retreat be accessible? If it is, will you be able to live in it?
- Are there plenty of trees and firewood?
- Is wild game available?

- Are there any natural sources of water nearby? Is it potable? Are there fish that can be caught?
- How likely is it that people driving by will see the retreat? Is it on a busy road that will see lots of traffic? Are there any major highways or thoroughfares nearby?
- How difficult will it be to defend the property from intruders should you be discovered?
- How hard is it going to be to get to the property if all major roads and highways are blocked or jammed?
- How close are you to densely populated areas?
- Could you walk to this location within 72 hours?

I have several locations mapped out that I can escape to. The first one is in the hills within a half hour of my house. I wouldn't head to this location if travel on the highway was still possible, but it's somewhere I could walk to in half a day if the highways were blocked and we had to set off on foot. The next location is in the same direction, but is a couple hours away. This is my ideal location because it's a cabin that's off the beaten path and it's unlikely anyone is going to stumble upon it. If they did, the dogs would alert me long before they made it to the door.

I have a third spot picked out even further away in case I'm forced to leave the second spot for some reason. This spot is even further off the beaten path and I would have to hike in to it, but it's a great choice if I want to get as far away from civilization as possible.

So, how will you know if it's time to head to your secondary retreat? There are many things that need to be considered. If you're living in a heavily populated area and it looks like the rule of law is crumbling, it's time to get out of there. If the food supply chain breaks down and store shelves are empty for more than a couple days, people are going to be desperate for food and will start looking elsewhere. Packs of armed and potentially-infected people will start searching house-to-house for food. Your home could become a target and you'll either have to fight off the bandits or sneak out the back door while they're raiding your home. It's better to gather your supplies and get out of the city while the getting's good because you'll have a giant target on your back if you're trying to leave with supplies in tow after the rule of law has broken down.

Once you've chosen your secondary retreat (and hopefully a couple more places you can escape to), it's time to sit down and map out multiple routes. The most important routes you're going to need to know are a number of ways you can get out of town and get headed in the right direction. Hop on Google Maps and look for smaller country roads and backroads you can use to get out of town. Dirt roads will be less-traveled, but they may be inaccessible in the winter unless you have a four wheel drive and even then they may not be safe. Map out as many routes as you can find and then drive the roads to see what they're like.

You may find that some of the roads you found on the map are private roads and they're gated off. These roads may be a good option when you're looking to get out of town because they won't be gridlocked. Don't cut the lock when you're checking out your routes, but keep a pair of bolt cutters in your vehicle that can be used to cut locks in an emergency.

The Bug Out Bag

The chances of Ebola striking so quickly you don't have time to gather supplies and get out of town is slim-to-none, but it's still a good idea to have a bag with a 72-hour supply of gear, food and other supplies packed and ready to go in case you need to get out of the house in a hurry. This type of bag is known as a bug out bag in the prepper and survival community. I recommend packing a bag for each family member who's old enough to carry one. I even have a small backpack for my 7-year old. It doesn't have a lot of stuff in it, but every little bit counts.

Entire books have been written about bug out bags, so it's going to be tough to cover everything in a chapter, but here are some of the items you're going to want to have in bag:

- **Food.** Here's where those MREs and freeze dried foods can be of benefit. They're small and light and a bunch of them will fit into a bug out bag without taking up too much space.
- **A basic first aid kit.**
- **A cell phone.**
- **A compass.**
- **A small wind-up radio.**
- **Fire starters.**
- **Flashlights and batteries.**
- **Lighters and fuel.**
- **Maps of your planned escape routes.**
- **Mess kits.**

- Mylar blankets.
- Personal documents.
- Sleeping bags.
- Tampons.
- Tent.
- Toilet paper.
- Utensils.
- **Warm clothing in winter and cool clothing in summer.**
- Water purification tablets or filters.
- Water.

Don't forget to pack enough medications to last you until you can get to a pharmacy. While a 72-hour supply of the items above is recommended, it's a good idea to have more than a 72-hour supply of prescription medications in your bag, especially if running out of the medications could be life-threatening. You never know when you'll have to leave town for an extended period of time and having extra medications will help ease the worry that you're going to run out of medicine and get sick.

Body Disposal

Whenever possible, let the professionals handle the disposal of human remains. The information in this chapter should only be used if there are no body disposal services available and the rule of law has broken down. Disposing of a body yourself is illegal in pretty much all jurisdictions, so keep this in mind if you decide to take matters into your own hands.

The key thing to remember is that the Ebola virus remains in the body for a long time after a victim dies. What this means is any body fluids you come in contact with can still infect you hours after the patient has succumbed to Ebola.

The CDC recommends that postmortem care personnel wear the following protective gear when handling bodies:

- **Face shield.**
- **Facemask.**
- **Impervious gown with full sleeves.**
- **Shoe covers.**
- **Surgical cap.**
- **Surgical scrub suit.**
- **Two pairs of surgical gloves.**

Leg coverings, aprons and other protective gear is optional, but encouraged. Think of it this way. The more layers of protection you have on. The less likely it becomes that there will be an accident where body fluids come in contact with bare skin.

Put the gear on before entering the room. It should be left on the entire time you're in the room. Wrap the body in plastic and place it into a leakproof bag if you have one available. If not, wrap the body in multiple layers of plastic and tape it shut in order to prevent fluids from leaking out. Keep your protective gear on while you carry the bag out of the house and only remove it once you're clear of the area where the body was left. Take care not to touch the outside of the gear while removing it. Wash your hands thoroughly with soap and water and incinerate the gear when you're done.

If possible, coordinate the transport of the remains with local and/or state authorities.

Addendum: Another Infection in New York

Things are moving so quickly with Ebola that it's difficult to keep up. Moments before this book was getting ready to go to press, another case of Ebola was announced in New York City.

It appears this is an isolated case occurring in a doctor who was recently working in an area of Africa where Ebola is found. He came down with a fever and gastrointestinal symptoms and notified the hospital and New York City Department of Health and Mental Hygiene. He was taken to the hospital by a team of trained specialists.

The people he came in contact with since arriving in America are being monitored, but so far it appears no one has caught the disease from the doctor. This is actually encouraging, since it provides at least anecdotal evidence that incidental contact with an infected person isn't going to result in infection. In all of the recent cases, a number of people have been in contact with the infected people and the only people to catch the Ebola virus on this continent have been two nurses tasked with caring for the first sick man to come into the country.

www.ingramcontent.com/pod-product-compliance
Lightning Source LLC
Chambersburg PA
CBHW071800170526
45167CB00003B/1110